Phosphorus, The Best Brain Food

"The Neglected Mineral That Makes You Smarter"

I0415482

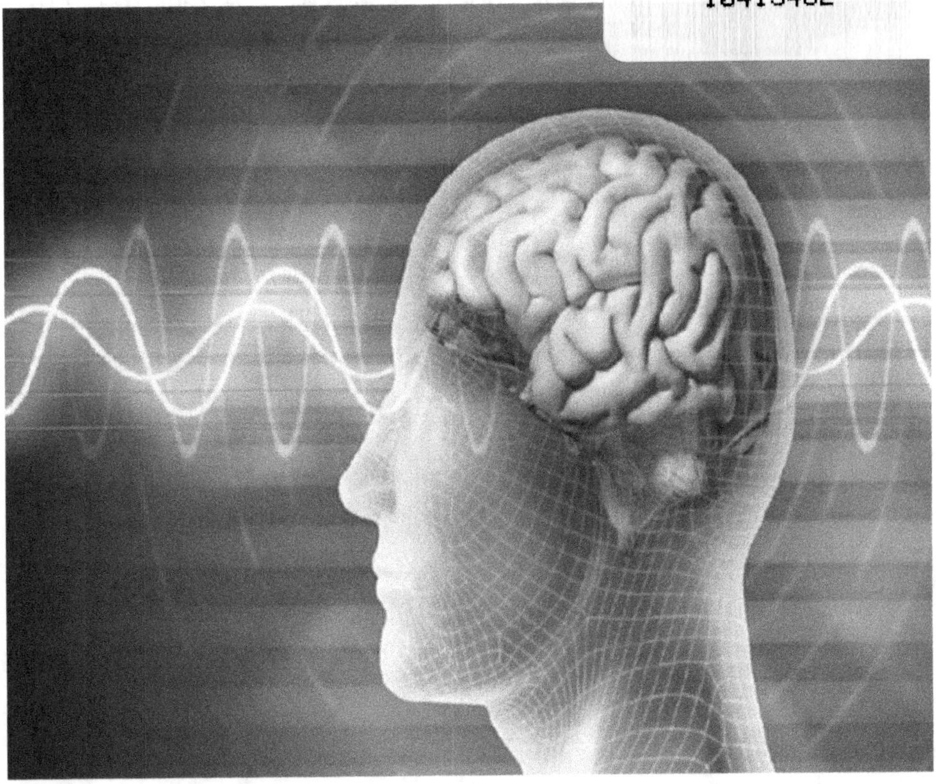

Rudy S. Silva, Natural Nutritionist

Table of Contents

Chapter 1: What Is Phosphorus All About?

If you want to have a top thinking brain, you will want to know the information in this book. What you need to know is that you don't want to be caught with a deficiency in phosphorus or an excess. You need to strive to keep a good balance of phosphorus because without a balance, many body functions are affected and the proper level of other minerals is decreased.

Phosphorus is the second highest mineral you have in your body. Eight-five percent of it is found in your bones and teeth. The other 15% is found in your RNA, DNA and other places in your body. It is a mineral that is necessary for the maintenance and growth of all the cells and tissues in your body. It also has a role in energy production boosting fatigue, muscle weakness, and bone fragility.

Phosphorus is a Macro mineral

Phosphorus is part of the seven macrominerals – calcium, sodium, potassium, magnesium, chlorine, and sulfur. The remaining minerals are called trace minerals and there are over 50 of them. Even though some of the trace minerals are micro amounts in our body, they have a function in keeping you healthy.

When you find that you are deficient in a mineral, you can eat more foods that contain that mineral or you supplement with that mineral. However, it not a good idea just to take a single mineral supplement or vitamin, since minerals and vitamins work together in a synergistic manner. Vitamins and minerals work as catalysts promoting the absorption and assimilation of other vitamins and minerals.

If you want to correct a mineral deficiency, then you need to take a supplement of that mineral in combination with other minerals to clear that deficiency. To compensate for a deficiency, at the start, you may have to take double or triple the dose listed on the bottle. After a week or two or even a month, you can go back to the maintenance dose on the bottle.

One of the best ways to take minerals and vitamins is to take them with food. In this fashion, the supplement you are taking can get the other vitamins or minerals it needs to be processed through your body properly.

Taking Phosphorus

The biological form of phosphorus is called phosphate. Phosphorus and phosphate may be used interchangeably in this book.

When you take a phosphorus supplement, you also need to take calcium, iron, manganese, sodium, and B6. So how do you do that? You need to take phosphorus or any mineral supplement with food.

It is important that all minerals used by your body be in balance. When you have too much or too little of any mineral, your health will be affected. It is the function of your elimination channels to get rid of the excess minerals and it is your job to take care of mineral deficiencies.

What Does Phosphorus Do In Your Body?

Here is what phosphorus does in your body. In your blood, it is needed for blood clotting. It is used to form teeth and bone. In your heart, it is needed for contractions and to keep your heart beating normal. Your cells use it for cell growth, creating energy, and it is needed for kidney function. Phosphorus helps your body to use vitamins and converts food into energy.

Brain

All parts of your brain depend on phosphorus to function properly – nerve networks, nervous system, and ganglia. High levels of thinking depend on phosphorus – psychic perceptions, idealistic thinking, and humanitarianism. With sulfur and omega fats, phosphorus vitalizes and regenerates your brain and nerves.

Without phosphorus you could not read, reason, create, visualize, study, memorize or comprehend. Is this a mineral you want to be caught short on?

Chapter 2: How Phosphorus Keeps You Alive

"Phosphorous is an essential brain nutrient"

Phosphorous is the major negative charged ion that exists throughout your body. Around 86 % of it is found in your bones and teeth, 13 % is in your soft tissue, and around 1% exists in the liquid outside of your cells, extracellular fluid. Outside the body, it is a highly toxic, nonmetallic, yellowish white element, which is insoluble in water, does not conduct electricity and has a low melting point of 110 deg F.

In your body phosphorous exist mostly **as a phosphate** ion in the following inorganic combination:

- Calcium phosphate

- Sodium phosphate

- Magnesium phosphate

- Iron phosphate

- Potassium phosphate

In this book, when we use the word phosphorus, it refers to one of the phosphate ions that are used in the condition we are talking about.

Your body contains around two pounds of phosphorus.

Aside from working with calcium to create bone structures, phosphorus also supports reactions with B vitamins, nerve, and muscle movement, cell division, transmitting hereditary traits, and digestion of food products at the cell level.

Here are the major functions of phosphorous:

- Makes up part of your cell membrane as phospholipids
- Holds DNA and RNA together
- Coats nerves of the brain
- Involved in muscle activity
- Assists in the brain and neurologic functions
- Used in brain cells and acts as a tonic for the brain and nerves
- Maintains higher intelligence and promotes idealistic ideas
- Involved in carbohydrate, protein, and fat metabolism
- Involved in the production of cell energy, ATP
- Primary ingredient in red blood cells
- Assist in buffering of acids and bases
- Works in white blood cell phagocytosis and platelet functions
- Combines with calcium to form and repair bone matrix
- Improves the reproduction systems
- Helps to maintain the body's pH levels
- Used to form new tissue and hair.
- Helps in forming the structure of teeth

Because phosphorus is heavily involved in building bones, it important that children get the required amount.

Phosphorus and Your Brain

One of the greatest functions of phosphorus is to help you maintain a high level of thinking. Phosphorous is burned up during heavy mental activity, such as concentration, hard studying, long and intense mental work, excess fears, drudgery, excessive drive to make money or succeed or to be better than the next person.

When you use up phosphorus, the phosphate wastes must be eliminated by the liver. It has been found that if you do a lot of mental activity, you will have more phosphorus in your urine than normal. With this type of loss, you need to make sure you are getting plenty of phosphorus in your diet.

If you are a student at any level, you need phosphorus every day. If you don't get phosphorus, your brain softens, wilts, and decays. Neuralgia develops and intelligence disappears.

To become more intelligent and have higher levels of thinking you need to have the highest levels of phosphorus in your body, without it affecting the balance of other minerals.

What is Lecithin?

Phosphorus is needed to produce lecithin, which is a complex fatty nutrient that you must have in your body. Without lecithin, you will become impotent, will get neuratrophia, will experience brain decomposition, have feeblemindedness, and have low nerve vitality. Taking lecithin daily in your diet helps to lessen the use of phosphorus and make it available for brain nutrition.

There are two types of phosphorous, one for the high level of thinking your brain does and the other for building bones.

Types of Phosphorus Food

The type of phosphorus that you need for bones come from vegetables and fruits and what we need for the brain and nervous system must come from eggs, meat, fish, chicken, turkey, other birds, and dairy. It is animal products that contain lecithin, which is a fat that carries the phosphorus and nutrients the brain needs. Phosphorus from meat carries a high vibrational frequency that is needed by your brain.

Vegetables do not have lecithin and carry a low amount of phosphorous, which is not enough for the body's needs.

Since the brain works at a faster speed, it uses a phosphorous that is capable of working at the speed of light. This is why brain phosphorous must come from animal meat, which vibrates at a higher frequency than vegetable phosphorous.

The word **Lecithin** comes from Greek, which means egg yolk. It is a fatty compound that is needed throughout your body. It is contained in the cell membrane, nerve tissue, brain, bile, semen, white and red blood corpuscles, lymph and serous fluids, and blood. Lecithin cannot be produced by your body, so you need to provide it through your food or by supplementation.

The phosphorescent glow many insects, fish, and other animals have, comes from the large quantities of phosphorous they contain. The energy the phosphorous molecule captures from outside itself allows it to release light or photons when activated. and in doing so it provides the energy for the brain to do its work at the speed of light. As light is released in your brain, your head would appear to glow, if you were sensitive enough to see the millions of small emissions of light going on all of the time.

Without phosphorous, we could not reason or comprehend. As you think and as information is being sent to different parts of your body, phosphorous is being used by your brain.

Research has shown that after excessive mental exertion phosphates are broken down, processed by the liver and kidney and show up as excess phosphorous in the urine.

Body Regulation of Phosphorous

The amount of phosphorous that your body maintains is based on:

- What you eat
- Your hormonal regulation
- What your kidney excretes through urine

After your Jejunum absorbs phosphorous and circulates it in your blood, your kidneys eliminate up to 90% of it, if necessary. Your gastrointestinal tract excretes the rest. Your gastrointestinal tract starts at your mouth and ends at your anus. So if you increase the amount of phosphorous foods or supplements you eat, your kidney adjusts the amount of phosphorus your body keeps.   But, if you lack phosphorous, your kidneys – nephrons - reabsorb phosphorous from the proximal tubules in an effort to bring phosphorous levels back to normal.

Nephron means kidney and is the basic structural and functional section of the kidney.   Its major function is to regulate the amount of water and various minerals your body needs by filtering your blood and excreting what your body does not need.

A nephron cleans your blood by eliminating blood waste and contaminates.   It regulates blood volume, pressure, electrolytes, metabolites, and pH.   The nephron is regulated by the endocrine system hormones – parathyroid hormone, antidiuretic hormone, and aldosterone.

The parathyroid gland also controls the level of phosphorous in your body.   It does this by monitoring the calcium level by controlling the parathyroid hormone, PTH since calcium and phosphorous must exist in your body in a certain ratio.   When calcium levels drop, phosphorous levels must increase.   PTH is released by the parathyroid causing an increase in calcium and phosphorous, which is obtained from your bones.   Suppressing the PTH activity causes deposition of calcium and phosphorous back into the bones.

Phosphorous levels are also increased by calcitriol that is found in your intestinal walls, which helps phosphorous to easily pass through the intestines.   Calcitriol is activated vitamin D, which is really a hormone and not a vitamin.   The vitamin D that is created on the skin goes through several chemical changes to become calcitriol or activated vitamin D.

It is this form of vitamin D that is attracted to the intestinal walls where it assists calcium and phosphorous to quickly and easily pass into your bloodstream.

If too much phosphorous accumulates in the lymph and blood, the kidney, acted upon by the PTH, increase the excretion of phosphorous through the urine. Low levels of PTH allow the kidney to reabsorb phosphorous from the blood instead of excreting it.

Phosphorous levels can also be depleted or changed by moving in and out of cells. In the case of alkalosis, - body liquids and blood exceed a pH of 7.4 alkalinity - phosphorous is used to drop down the pH in cells and in the blood. Also when insulin moves into the cells to carry in glucose, it also drags in phosphorous causing the extracellular fluid to become more alkaline. So the amount of insulin activity in cells also affects the levels of phosphorous.

Hypophosphatemia (Insufficient Phosphorus)

Hypophosphatemia happens when the serum phosphorus level falls below 1.8mEq/L. Serum phosphorus refers to the amount of this element in your blood plasma, which is that part of the blood that is clear, sticky and contains no blood cells, platelets, or fibrinogen. If your serum phosphorus level falls below 0.8 mEq/L, your body would not have the energy to provide organ function.

How do you get to the point where you lack phosphorous in your body? There are at least four ways.

- Movement of phosphorous in cell structure

- Decrease of phosphorous adsorption

- Decrease kidney reabsorption
- Lack of phosphorus from diet

The movement of **phosphorus from an extracellular** liquid into intracellular liquid occurs under many conditions. This happens during hyperventilation, alcohol withdrawal, heat stroke, pain, anxiety, diabetic ketoacidosis, and acute salicylate poisoning. When you have excess glucose in your blood, the pancreas releases insulin to remove this excess and move it into your cells. In this process, insulin moves glucose into your cells but it also moves phosphorous with it.

When phosphorous is moved into your cells, the phosphorous levels outside the cells fall and phosphorous from the blood is released to rebalance this loss. But then blood phosphorous drops and needs to be replaced by your bones, food, or wherever it can be found in your body.

When you have poor adsorption or are starved, your body phosphorous levels will drop. When you use antacids or sucralfate – a drug for ulcers - they bind with phosphorous and decrease it below normal levels. Use of laxative can also cause excess phosphorous to be excreted in feces. Lack of vitamin D is another cause of phosphorous not being absorbed. Vitamin D in the intestine is necessary to pull phosphorous through the intestinal walls.

The following drugs can bind with phosphorus and decrease its movement into your body:

- Acetazolamide
- Thiazide diuretics
- Chlorothiazide

- Hydrochlorothiazide
- Loop diuretics
- Bumetanide
- Furosemide
- Antacids
- Aluminum carbonate
- Aluminum hydroxide
- Calcium carbonate
- Magnesium oxide
- Insulin
- Laxatives

Use of diuretics is the most common cause of phosphorous loss through the kidneys. People with diabetic ketoacidosis and poor control of blood glucose levels have increased urine output, causing loss of phosphorous. Burn victims also exhibit a high loss of phosphorous. This may be a result of excess urination.

Chapter 3: Sicknesses From Insufficient Phosphorus

Hypophosphatemia

When you lack phosphorus, it's called hypophosphatemia and typically it's a result from a poor diet or from a catabolic state where you exercise too much or when you fast or go without food for a long time. If you drink too much alcohol, you probably are low in phosphorus.

Here are some more reasons why you might low in phosphorus.

- Intestinal malabsorption
- Chronic diarrhea
- Hypomagnesemia
- Deficient in vitamin D – necessary for phosphorus absorption
- Chronic use of antacids
- Kidney tubular defects
- Diabetic acidosis
- Injured cells releasing phosphorus

Here are a few symptoms of Hypophosphatemia:

If you are suffering from lack of phosphorous, your body will exhibit a variety of symptoms. You will have:

- Anxiety
- Anorexia
- Low tissue oxygenation
- Constant faintness
- Lack of appetite or extreme hunger
- Weak sexual system
- Nerve pain
- Difficulty reasoning with headaches
- Entire nervous system is weak
- Mental states go from apprehension to laughter
- Mood changes from happiness to sadness
- Emotional needs increase: love, affection, acceptance, sympathy, and acknowledgment
- Bone deformations
- Poor blood formation
- Muscle weakness
- Tremors
- Impaired red blood cell functions
- Irregular breathing
- Numbness
- Stiff joints

Personality changes occur rapidly from calmness to hysteria. Your brain does not function well and confusion dominates. Night time brings fear and depression. Any noises disturb you. You become disgusted with yourself and those around you. Your choice of foods changes and you dislike foods you once liked. You develop a lack of confidence.

Bone deformations

If you lack phosphorus, you will not be able to properly grow bones. It is associated with rickets in children and osteomalacia, softening of bones, in adults.

Blood

Phosphorus plays a role in the formation of red, white blood cells, and platelets. Lack of phosphorus affects the amount of red blood cells that form and this, in turn, affects the amount of oxygen your cells receive.

Here are the RDA phosphorus **daily requirements.**

Age	RDA Phosphorus Requirements
Pregnant- Breastfeeding	1200 mg
Birth to 6 months	100 mg
7 to 12 months	275 mg
1 to 3 years	460mg
4 to 8 years	500 mg
9 to 18 years	1250 mg

19 years and above   700 mg

Chapter 4: Sicknesses From Excess Phosphorus

Hyperphosphatemia

Hyperphosphatemia occurs when your serum phosphorus level exceeds 2.6mEq/L when your kidneys can not excrete your excess phosphorous or when damage cells spill out excess phosphorous. An increase in dietary phosphorous can also cause Hyperphosphatemia. And, if you overuse laxatives that contain phosphates or do phosphate enemas, you will have an increase of phosphorus in your body.

Sodas

Sodas have a high quantity of phosphorus. The danger of drinking a lot of sodas is that your phosphorus levels will increase and this will affect the level of body calcium. Phosphorus and calcium balance each other in your body and work together to build bones. Excess phosphorus decreases your calcium levels by binding or combining with it.

In this case, to decrease your phosphorus levels, you need to decrease your soda intake to one a day or none at all.

Another issue is that phosphorus also binds with magnesium, manganese, zinc, and copper, which infers with the work these minerals need to do.

So, don't drink regular, caffeine-free, diet, and club soda.

Protein

When you eat meat, you lose calcium. Since meat is acidic, calcium is used to neutralize this acid and in doing so affects the balance of phosphorus. If you don't have enough calcium in your body stores, calcium will be pulled from your bones.

Meat protein is more acidic than the protein in fish, nuts, seeds, beans, and dairy products so less calcium is lost when you eat these foods.

The **kidneys** are responsible for most of the phosphorous excretion. They usually excrete the same amount that is absorbed through the digestive system. But, when they don't, your body has more phosphorous than it needs. When the thyroid or parathyroid is damage or malfunctions, PTH hormone, which regulates phosphorous excretion from the kidney, is decreased causing an increase in phosphorous in your body.

The transcellular shift of phosphorous in cells, movement of phosphorus in and out of your cells, can cause a rise in body phosphorous levels. Here is a list of problems that can cause transcellular shifts.

- Acid-base imbalances
- Cellular destruction
- Chemotherapy

- Muscle necrosis
- Infections
- Heat stroke
- Trauma

An excess intake of phosphorous also increases body phosphorous. This increase can come from the excess use of phosphorous or vitamin D supplements, laxatives, and enemas.

One problem that can cause by Hyperphosphatemia is a decrease in calcium or hypocalcemia since these minerals have an inverse relationship, an increase in one follows a decrease in the other. This results in bone weakness or osteoporosis. In acute Hyperphosphatemia, the symptoms are usually caused by hypocalcemia, loss of calcium.

Symptoms of Hyperphosphatemia:

- Osteoporosis
- Seeks out psychics-palm readers, wants to know about his future
- Feels he is superior and more knowledgeable
- Excessive expression or happy emotions
- Overworks his mind
- Detest daily routine matters

Tends toward occult subjects, spiritual and mystical

activities.

Chapter 5: Phosphorus Foods For Your Brain

Foods for Your Brain

When you lack phosphorous in your body the best way to correct this deficiency is through diet, eating high phosphorous foods, and through supplementation. The body always knows how much phosphorus and other minerals it needs. So any excess you take in, your body will excrete it, if your body is healthy.

The highest foods in phosphorous, for your brain, are:

Meat, egg yolk, fish, dairy products, Cottage cheese, Beef Liver, dried fruits, Swiss cheese, sardines

The highest foods in phosphorous for bone building are:

Almonds, rice bran, wheat bran, pumpkin, squash, seeds, lentils, soybeans, sunflower seeds, soybeans, flaxseeds, navy and pinto beans, oats, quinoa,

Here is an additional list of high phosphorous foods:

Almonds, barley, bass, lentils, Beans, milk, millet, oats, Fish, bone broth, cabbage, olives, Cardamom, pecans, carrots, cashews, Cheese, rice bran, rye, sardines, Cod roe, corn, Dulse, sole, Trout, real butter, halibut, haddock, Artichoke

Meat

Meat contains 22 times more phosphorus than calcium, so this creates a nutritional imbalance since your body needs both these minerals in the same amounts. When you have an excess of phosphorus, it will deplete that calcium in your body. The reason is that calcium is needed to digest phosphorus.

When you are not low in phosphorus, it is best not to load up on meat. Eating too much meat can cause deficiencies in vitamin B6, vitamin B3, and magnesium. In addition, your body produces ammonia after metabolizing meat. It has been found that ammonia is a dangerous carcinogen and one of the causes of colon cancer. So for a good diet, eat small amounts of meat and eat plenty of nuts, fruits, and vegetables.

Nuts

One of the overall great foods to eat is nuts and almonds. They should be at the top of your list for phosphorus. The phosphorus they contain in 2/3 cup is 475mg. Use a variety of nuts as snacks and in food. Use peanuts or smooth peanut butter for phosphorus. Other nuts to use are almonds, cashews, pecans, sunflower seeds and walnuts.

Whole Flaxseeds

Flaxseeds are high in omega-3, which benefit your brain and heart. These seeds contain lignans which an antioxidant which helps in all kinds of inflammation.

Ground up 2 tablespoons of flaxseeds and add them to your smoothies, cereals, or unsweetened yogurt. Add a bit of honey to your yogurt.

Milk and Yogurt

Milk and unsweetened yogurt are a good source of phosphorus and they also contain calcium, vitamin D, magnesium, and protein.

Low Fat Cheese and Cottage cheese

Low Fat Cheese and Cottage cheese are a good source of phosphorus. Use the Blue, feta, and Gouda cheese. Many nutritionists feel that a high-fat content cheese can decrease your absorption of calcium. However, cottage cheese has a good ratio of calcium to phosphorus that makes this a great balanced mineral food.

Bran

Oat, wheat, and rice bran are a rich source of phosphorus. Eat bran every day by putting them in your smoothies, salads, and cereals. Bran is a high source of fiber and will help you keep you free of illness.

Beef Liver

Beef liver is also very high in phosphorus. Eating 3 1/2 oz. of beef liver gives you 476 mg of phosphorus. Eat only organic liver or range liver, since other types of liver may have too many toxins.

Vegetables

Broccoli is a great source of phosphorus compared to other greens. In addition, it is also rich in antioxidants and vitamin C.Eat beans and peas for their source of phosphorus.

Sodas

Sodas are so popular that many people can't eat their meal without them. Sodas do not have any health benefits and any energy boost you get from them comes from the sugar and caffeine that they have.

Because sodas have high phosphorus content, they may and probably interfere with your calcium absorption. Their sugar and phosphoric acid that they contain can lead to weight gain and tooth decay. Read the soda label so that you know what you are drinking. Most colas and pepper flavored sodas contain a large amount of phosphorus. For children, this could result in restlessness or sleepiness. Children should not drink sodas and adults should use them sparingly.

Here is the quantity of phosphorus in the best sources of phosphorus foods in mg.

- Soybeans   one cup 1309
- Flaxseeds....................one Tbs 65.8
- Lentils   one cup 866
- Navy beans...................one cup 846
- Oats   one cup 816

- Pinto beans.........................one cup 793

- Quinoa   one cup 777

- Swiss cheese.......................one slice 159

- Sardines   one sardine 59

- Dried peas.........................one cup 721

- Lima Beans   one cup 685

- Sesame Seeds...................one cup 986

- Rye   one cup 632

- Brown Rice.........................one cup 185

- Peanuts   one cup 523

- Barley.............................one cup 486

- Almonds   one oz 137

- Eggs...............................one medium egg 84

- Atlantic Salmon   one-half fillet 449

- Tempeh............................one cup 442

- Chicken   one half chicken breast 196

- Sunflower seeds.................one cup 304

- Garbanzo Beans   one cup 276

- Tuna...................................one can 269

- Kidney beans   one cup 244

- Tofu....................................one half cup 239

- Yogurt   .   one cup 233

- Potatoes.............................one large potato

- Cod   one fillet 202

- Fresh peas.........................one cup 187

Eat a variety of these foods. If you need higher levels of thinking and clarity, eat more of the food higher in phosphorus and use a phosphorus supplement.

Chapter 6: Phosphorus Supplements

Food can supply you with plenty of phosphorus. It is ok to take phosphorus supplements, but do not use in place of food.

Typically, you don't need to take a supplement for phosphorus, since foods can supply plenty of it. But, if you find that you need to supplement with phosphorus, here is some information to consider.

Do not take phosphorus supplements with potassium supplements. Phosphorus will interact with potassium resulting in excess potassium in your blood leading to heart issues.

When you take mineral supplements, you want them to be "chelated." What this means is that the mineral in question is chemically bonded to an amino acid. In the food you eat, minerals always combine with an amino acid. Your body recognizes chelated minerals and absorbs them quickly and easily. This is why fresh juices are so good because they contain minerals in chelated form.

When you have severe hypophosphatemia you will require an I.V. infusion of potassium phosphate. This is the fastest way to get phosphorus into your body.

Phosphorus Dose

Young adults aged 11 to 24 should have 1200mg of phosphorus daily. Children from 1 to 10 years require 500 to 800mg daily. Typically, you would get this phosphorus from the food you eat.

The adult daily recommendation for phosphorous is 800 to 1200 mg, which is easily absorbed through the Jejunum.

The Jejunum is part of the small intestine and the part that follows the duodenum. The small intestine consists of the duodenum, jejunum, and ileum. The duodenum is the part that is attached to the stomach. The section passed the duodenum is called the jejunum.

When the stomach content is processed it moves into the duodenum where the majority of this food is absorbed. The jejunum is the center of the small intestine and the ileum is the last part, which is attached to the large intestine or ascending colon.

Phosphorus Supplements

Homeopathic supplements

Neutra-Phos or Neutra-PhosX- Each tablet contains 852 mg dibasic sodium phosphate anhydrous, 155 mg monobasic potassium phosphate, and 130 mg monobasic sodium phosphate monohydrate. Each tablet yields approximately 250 mg of phosphorus, 298 mg of sodium (13.0 mEq) and 45 mg of potassium (1.1 mEq). This product can purchased on the internet. You should consult with your doctor before taking this supplement.

Natrum Phos.6x – is a homeopathic supplement and can be purchased at most health food stores.

Weleda Phosphorus 30C

Weleda phosphorus 30C is also a homeopathic remedy. It is useful for a cough, hoarseness, night sweats, and sleeplessness. It should only be taken for a short period.

Lecithin

You can buy lecithin in granule form or in capsules. It is best to take it in granule form. You can add it to your salads, soups, cereal, or other food you like. You can use a tablespoon each time you use it. It has little taste and it is soft. Keep it in your refrigerator to keep it fresh.

Phosphorous is a creator of light in the body and promotes intellect, thinking, higher reasoning, and abstract thoughts. It is a brain nutrient and is brought into the brain by lecithin which is found in meat, egg yolk and fish. It improves nerve function and brain nutrition.

It is also active in creating a bone matrix and this phosphorous comes from fruits and vegetables. It affects muscle tissue and is necessary for sexual function and reproduction.

Bone Meal

Bone meal is a good source of phosphorus and comes in tablets or powder. Look for bone meal that is raw, unheated, and from South America. Use tablets per day or 1/2 tablespoon.

Phosphorus Liquid provided by ProCelleHealth

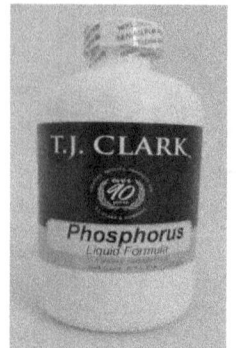

Phosphorus liquid is an ionic supplement that is bio-available and is quickly absorbed by your body. Taking 10 drops provides 45 mg of phosphorus. This is considered professional grade phosphorus. It can be added to juices or water.

Even though you take supplements, not all of the phosphorus in these supplements will be absorbed into your body. Some of this phosphorus may be used up in your stomach, or pass right by the small intestine, and into your colon to be excreted.

CHAPTER 7: The Best Way To Power Up Your Brain

Powering up your brain is not just about one mineral, phosphorus, but about the combination of minerals, nutrients, and lifestyle. But, for sure without the proper amount of phosphorus, your mental abilities will suffer.

Here are some other ideas and supplements that you need to consider for maximizing your overall brain function.

- Inflammation
- Acid body
- Anxiety
- Exercise
- Supplements

Inflammation

If you have inflammation in your body, this inflammation is reflected in your brain and your brain has to respond or prepare for how this inflammation will affect it. This brain response requires energy and focus and this takes away from your intellectual focus. Reducing your body inflammation will allow your brain to have more mental energy to make you more intelligent and resourceful.

When you are sick in any way, you can see that you cannot focus on intellectual ideas. You cannot focus on school or business studies at a high level. Most everyone has body inflammation, even if they don't detect it. This is called low-level inflammation that over time will create devastating disease. This low-level inflammation comes from unhealthy living habits that cause your body distress.

Acid Body

Having an acid body is not normal. The norm is an alkaline body. An acid body destroys body cells, tissue, and organs. This destruction is a result of inflammation. To minimize body inflammation, you need to be aware of how to reduce body acids. Acids accumulate in your body when you have a poor diet and eat plenty of junk food. You can reduce body acids and inflammation by eating more fruits and vegetables and getting away from junk food.

Anxiety

Anxiety creates acids and excessive anxiety produces an acid body. Anxiety always leads to inflammation which affects brain function. If you require high levels of thinking, then you have to determine what you need to do to reduce anxiety and stress.

There are many stress reduction programs. Ultimately, stress is caused by your own inability to adapt to ideas that run against your established opinion, education, and philosophy. It is up to you to unravel yourself so that you can begin to realize that your view of the world is but one reality. There is one book written by Arthur Janov called "Why You Get Sick." This book identifies where anxiety and stress originate.

Exercise

Exercise of any kind is necessary for maintaining good brain function. Exercise increases blood flow to your brain to deliver nutrients and remove toxic matter. It strengthens all parts of your body and improves your immune system, which allows you to fight off inflammation.

Supplements

The supplements that you need for keeping your brain sharp are listed below. You do not have to take all of these but you should use 2-3 of them and rotate to others after a few weeks or month.

Acetylcholine provides your brain with choline. It is choline that regulates cognitive function and memory. It protects your brain cells from free radical damage. It improves brain communication between cells. You can check out a product called **Brain Vitality Plus** which provides a pure source of choline.

Green tea has one of the highest levels of antioxidants. This tea is necessary for great body and brain health. Drink a cup two times a day with added grated ginger. You can add a touch of honey to make taste better.

Curcumin is a powerful anti-oxidant that has been found to reduce inflammation in all parts of the body. It is found in the spice turmeric but in little amounts. You can buy it in capsules so that you can receive its potential for improving your brain health.

The active form of curcumin is called 95% tetra-hydro curcuminoids. Using this form of curcumin allows your body to readily absorb it.

Curcumin is a fat-soluble compound that becomes more bioavailable when mixed with pepper or black seed oil.

Gingko biloba has been used to treat high blood pressure and vascular diseases. In many clinical studies, Ginkgo has been found to increase the blood flow rate in capillaries and end arteries. The action of Ginkgo is to neutralize the effects of free radicals.

These radicals are known for damaging the interior walls of veins and arteries. Damage to these walls causes the buildup of plaque, which then leads to poor blood flow to the brain and all parts of the body.

Ginger is also anti-inflammatory and increases blood circulation. It is easy to use by grating it and putting into a green tea.

Fish oil is a great benefit for your brain. It contains a great source of omega-3. It has anti-inflammatory properties and can bring more oxygen into your brain.

Lecithin will provide you with choline and phospholipids that are used by your brain for better brain cell communication.

Antioxidants help fight inflammation by neutralizing free radicals that are creating in your body or that are eaten. Free radicals are found personal body products, junk food, and in the water or air, you breathe.

All fruits and vegetables are high in antioxidants. Some are higher than others, but eating the different color produce will assure that you get a variety of antioxidants.

Coconut is a brain food. Your brain survives on glucose but there is another food that your brain uses to live on. Your brain thrives on medium chain fatty acids (MCF.) It is these MCFs that can pass your blood-brain barrier to provide the food your brain needs. If you're glucose resistance where your body has a hard time passing glucose into your cells, then your brain can use MFCs for brain food.

Use all parts of the coconut for better brain function; coconut water, milk, coconut meat, coconut oil, coconut oil supplements, and MCF coconut.

Digestive enzymes help you digest your food. If you suffer from acid reflux, bloating, digestive problems, or constipation, you should be taking digestive enzymes. It is of great benefit to provide your digestive system with enzymes. A poor digestive system contributes to a variety of body inflammation.

Aside from digestive enzymes capsules, eating pineapples and papayas can provide with some digestive enzymes.

Cacao is high flavonoids, which have antioxidant properties. Antioxidants protect cells and tissue from free radical damage, which results in inflammation. Theobromine is found in cacao which increases neurotransmitter activity giving you a mood elevation. Eat the cacao in chocolate that has 70 to 80 % cacao that is sweetened with stevia.

By concentrating on more phosphorus foods, supplements and the ideas presented above, you can power up your brain beyond what you thought was possible.

Chapter 8: About The Author And Other Resources

Rudy Silva is a natural consultant nutritionist educated in the United State of Nutrition and Physics. He is a graduate of the San Jose State University in California. He is the author of 30 other e-books on natural remedies. He has authored a newsletter in natural remedies for over 4 years. He has many websites promoting special recommended products and information.

Resource page

Here are some of the other books about natural remedies that have been written by this author. You can see the entire list at:

To see all of the books written by this author, go to this URL:

http://tinyurl.com/b2f7wd3

If you need support or want to promote any of his books, please contact him at rss41@yahoo.com and expect a reply within 24 hours. He looks forward to hearing from you and is happy to help you understand his material on natural and nutritional health.

Give A Review

And, don't forget to give a review for this book so that others can gain the benefits of what is in this e-book.

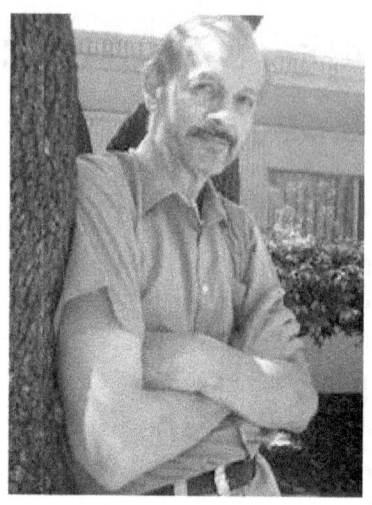

To you, for losing weight, creating better health and more happiness in your life,

Rudy S Silva